OFF THE COUCH

*How to Find Joy Through Physical
Activity Even If You Hate to Exercise*

Melissa Wogahn, MA

Off the Couch: How to Find Joy Through
Physical Activity Even If You Hate to Exercise

Publisher's Cataloging-In-Publication Data
(Prepared by The Donohue Group, Inc.)
Names: Wogahn, Melissa.
Title: Off the couch : how to find joy through physical activity even if
you hate to exercise / Melissa Wogahn, MA.
Description: Carlsbad, California : PartnerPress.org, [2017] | Includes
bibliographical references.
Identifiers: LCCN 2016921220 | ISBN 978-1-944098-00-1 (paperback)
| ISBN 978-1-944098-01-8 (ebook)
Subjects: LCSH: Exercise. | Physical fitness. | Exercise--Psychological
aspects. | Physical fitness--Psychological aspects. | Joy.
Classification: LCC RA781 .W64 2017 (print) | LCC RA781 (ebook) |
DDC 613.71--dc23

Additional worksheets are available for free by visiting
www.JoyOfActiveLiving.com/couch

Published by PartnerPress | Carlsbad, California

This book is available for bulk purchase or for private
label publishing by associations, corporate wellness
programs and other health and wellness organizations.
Please email **publish@partnerpress.org** for details.

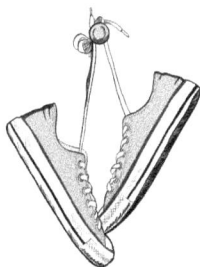

Contents

Introduction 1

What is an Active Life? 9
› Get Active and Help Your Brain......................... 10
› Granny Power.. 14

Create Your Active-Living Vision 19
› Be Clear on Why it is Important to You 23
› What do you value?... 23
› Knowledge is Power... 25
› Health Coaching 26
› Gain Perspective.. 27
› How Confident Do You Feel?............................. 28
› What are your challenges?................................... 29
› Abby—Getting active for an event, or for life? .. 30
› Stories That Inspire Us
› Patience: Your New Friend.................................. 35

Stages of Change: Your Key to Success 39
› Not Considering or Not Interested: Pre-
  Contemplation 40

› Contemplation, or, "I May Get Active"............. 42

› Preparation "I Will"... 43

› I Am Active: Action!... 44

› I Am Still Active! 45

› One Step at a Time to an Active Life 48

› Stage 1: Pre Contemplation 50

› Stage 2: Contemplation 53

› Stage 3: Preparation or "I Will".......................... 55

› Stage 4: I Am Active... 57

› Stage 5: I Am Still Active.................................... 61

› Tips for the Discouraged or Impatient Thinkers . 65

Goal Setting: Your Ticket to Success 69

› Carmine—Starting Small.................................... 72

› Stories That Inspire Us

› Early Stage Goals.. 74

› Cheryl—Learning to Adjust Goals 79

› Stories That Inspire Us

› Smart Goals... 81

Mindfulness 87

› Mindfulness Activity... 90

Activity Style Assessment 95

Resources 109

› Organizations.. 109

› Online resources (your tax dollars at work!)..... 110

› Apps.. 111

› Educational Documentaries.............................. 112

› Books 112

Notes.. 115

Acknowledgments 116

About the Author 117

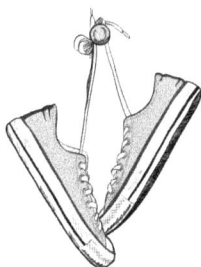

Introduction

"Sometimes the greatest challenge is to actually begin." —John O'Donohue

WHEN I WAS GROWING UP, I never really thought about physical activity. I was active enough; I was on a swim team as a young child and high school student. I had a horse that I rode every day, and I had to walk up steep hills to get to her corral. I used to challenge myself to see how fast I could make it to the top of the road. By the time I made it to the top, I was breathing heavily and sweating, and I remember loving that feeling.

Then I went away to college. I lived a typical college student lifestyle: stressful studying, eating lots of sugar carbohydrates, and not exactly living an active life. And, although I was a physical education major, I felt sorely out of shape. Then I was asked to teach a fitness class. Having taught swimming and gymnastics during high school, I knew that I enjoyed teaching. So I began a long tenure of group fitness instruction. In retrospect, I now see that teaching provided the opportunity for me to be active and that fit my next phase of life. Now, some thirty years later, I have had to adjust many times to different ways of living actively. And all I can say is that if I can do it, you can too. Even if you have never been active, you can grow into a life of activity on your own terms. What I know for sure is that living an active life is not a stop/start endeavor; it is a fluid process in which we continue to adapt.

A little history of how I came to write this book:

After completing my master's degree in exercise physiology, I began my postgraduate studies in a medical fitness setting where I oversaw program operations servicing more than 150 clients per day in a structured fitness/nutrition program. Clients participated in an hour of both physical activity and lifestyle education. This experience was transformative for me as I witnessed how physical activity can help people realize a better quality of life. I then had the good fortune to work in a variety of clinical settings. I worked with physicians, physical and occupational therapists, psychologists, and pain management specialists. I saw many sick, unconditioned, and injured people and I couldn't help but wonder why no one was addressing their poor physical condition. As an exercise physiologist, I wanted to advocate education programs to get sick and injured people more active, reduce further risk of injury, and increase their health and wellbeing. There was pushback from healthcare providers who believed that because insurance would not cover exercise education services, patients would not be motivated to move on their own. And quite frankly, with the healthcare model at the time, it was just too hard to advocate regular exercise for their patients.

Fast forward twenty-five years and we now have a healthcare system that spends between $147 and $200 billion dollars per year on obesity-related preventable diseases. Obesity is associated with job absenteeism costing nearly $4.3 billion annually. The good news is that due in large part to rising healthcare costs, the importance of physical activity for preventative health has finally gained acceptance. Dr. John Ratey, author of "Spark: The Revolutionary Science of Exercise and the Brain," states that, "The mechanisms by which exercise changes how we think and feel are so much more effective than donuts, medicines and wine." He goes on to state that "even 10 minutes of activity changes your brain."

There is a push for physicians to use physical activity as a vital sign similar to blood pressure and heart rate. Kaiser Permanente has instituted the *Exercise as a Vital Sign* initiative in which patients are asked two basic questions: how many days per week they engage in physical activity, and how many minutes they spend doing it. In 2007, the American College of Sports Medicine® and the American Medical Association® formed *Exercise is Medicine*, an organization dedicated to bridging the gap between physicians, patients and exercise professionals. Other organizations, including *Everybody Walk* and *Walk With A Doc*, are continuing to spread the message of physical activity and its impact on health and wellbeing.

The case is pretty clear that exercise can do wondrous things. But what if you hate to exercise?

Many people begin an exercise program only to stop after a few short months. Perhaps they get injured, bored, or just tired of all the work and attention that an active life requires. Or maybe they stop because they hate to move. What's missing is their platform for lasting change: in other words, they have not done the foundational inner work to set themselves up for long-term success.

This book is intended to help move you from an inactive life to a life of less depression, more energy, and a wealth of gosh-darn positive vibes. I believe that physical activity can be a springboard to a life full of possibility.

I want to make this point clear: this book doesn't tell you what activities to do. Rather, the exercises in this book put you in the driver's seat by providing tools to look within and finally figure out what kind of active life will work for you.

According to the Center for Disease and Control and Prevention, only 21% of adults meet the 2008 Physical Activity Guidelines for both aerobic and muscle-strengthening activity.[1] Thirty percent do no exercise at all. But steps are being taken to make it easier for people to live active lives. The federal government has launched an effort with state and local communities to construct environments with sidewalks and bike paths away from traffic. The US Department of Transportation has even developed a *Resident's Guide for Creating Safer Walking and Biking Communities*, a terrific resource for people interested in creating change to support an active environment. Workplace wellness programs have evolved over the years to encourage and support employees to make healthier choices. Along with a supportive environment, however, individuals need tools and insight to learn how to think actively.

This book will help develop a foundation for success by helping you discover why you want to live actively and why it is important to you. You will learn how to think differently about physical activity. Once you go from doing nothing to doing something, you will discover the joy of living an active life and become the best you can be.

1 | What is an Active Life?

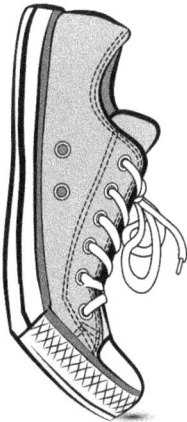

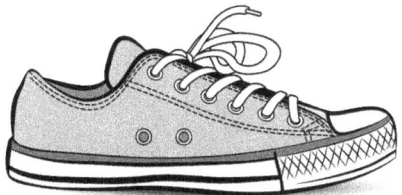

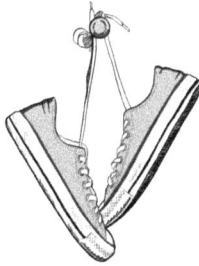

What is an Active Life?

AS ONE FITNESS JOURNALIST SURMISED, "Five years of fitness reporting and [one] lesson: just move."[2] There is a misconception among sedentary people that exercise has to be intense, painful and full of misery. An exercise session can be that, but it doesn't have to. Just move. It is no secret that physical activity makes us feel better. Exercise *is* medicine. I like to call it our own spoonful of sugar. Exercising regularly helps manage weight, control blood pressure, reduce stress, better sleep patterns, increase bone density, and basically make us feel better. According to the American College of Sports Medicine,

Regular physical activity can:

- Reduce mortality and the risk of recurrent breast cancer by approximately 50%.
- Lower the risk of colon cancer by over 60%.
- Reduce the risk of developing of Alzheimer's disease by approximately 40%.
- Reduce the incidence of heart disease and high blood pressure by approximately 40%.
- Lower the risk of stroke by 27%.
- Lower the risk of developing type II diabetes by 58%
- Be twice as effective in treating type II diabetes as the standard insulin prescription and save as much as $2250 per person per year when compared to the cost of standard drug treatment.
- Decrease depression as effectively as Prozac or behavioral therapy.

Miriam Nelson, PhD, Director of the John Hancock Research Center on Physical Activity, Nutrition and Obesity Prevention at Tufts University succinctly states, "We've yet to find a disease where exercise isn't helpful."

Get Active and Help Your Brain

Your brain loves physical activity and it is worth understanding how exercise can influence brain function and increase resiliency—our ability to handle difficult or stressful situations.

The resilience center of the brain is located in the prefrontal cortex. This is the area of the brain that is termed "the seat of executive functions," or the area responsible for how we interact with the outside world. The prefrontal cortex also receives messages from other parts of the brain having to do with emotions–namely, fear and anxiety. There are cells in the prefrontal cortex that secrete a neuropeptide which inhibits fear and calms us down. Resilient people have thirty times more activity in their prefrontal cortex! If you feel stressed and want tools to help manage stress, keep reading.

There are techniques that stimulate activity in the prefrontal cortex. These include meditation, affirmations, breathing exercises, and *physical activity*. Exercise stimulates prefrontal cortex activity, which calms us down, increases our resiliency, and improves our ability to deal with life's twists and turns. So instead of feeling as though we cannot cope, physical activity will give us a way out of the madness into the wondrous state of, "I am okay, life is good, and everything will work out."

Here is another great thing about exercise: physical activity increases serotonin and decreases cortisol. Serotonin, a neurotransmitter, is believed to be responsible for maintaining emotional balance. Cortisol is a stress hormone and when elevated is correlated with weight gain. And here is the good news: a little bit of exercise goes a long way. A 20-30 minute walk on most days of the week can lower cortisol. In looking at other benefits from the exercise/serotonin/cortisol connection, here are three more reasons to focus on exercise:

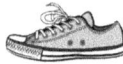

Exercise = Better Mood + Better Sleep + Increased Willpower

1. Willpower—Exercise can help increase willpower.
2. Food cravings—Exercise can decrease food cravings.
3. Exercise can improve sleep.

So regular exercise helps us eat better, sleep better and basically feel better about who we are.

This is important because how we react to daily occurrences has such a profound influence on how we feel about ourselves and the choices we make whether to support our intention to be active or succumb to a chaotic and out of control existence of sedentary living. Let exercise be your best friend who will always be there for you. So in addition to the physiological benefits of exercise, our brains benefit from activity, too. It can be another motivating factor to finally do something and get active.

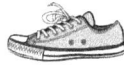

I tell people that going for a run is like taking a little bit of Prozac and a little bit of Ritalin because, like the drugs, exercise elevates these neurotransmitters. Exercise balances neurotransmitters—along with the rest of the neurochemicals in the brain. Keeping your brain in balance can change your life.

—John Ratey, MD, author of SPARK
and co-founder of Sparking Life

So what does all this mean? It's very simple. We don't need fancy equipment. We don't need snazzy clothes, makeup, or the latest fad DVD. We don't have to look good. Not ever. All we need to do is move. Period. It doesn't matter what we do, but do something—a little bit—every day. And don't worry about what others say.

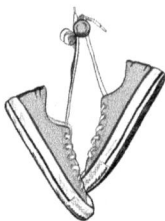

Stories That Inspire Us

THE SETTING IS A SOUTH AFRICAN township. The characters are old ladies. They play soccer. While appearing lumpy and bumpy and limping toward the ball, these ladies know the secret to life.

The group began with the loving intervention of a woman named Beka Ntsanwisi who has performed extensive work in the rural communities of South Africa. While working as a support network for sick ladies in the hospital, she introduced them to exercise. As a light-hearted joke, she suggested they play soccer.

These grannies, the oldest being 84, had significant health issues including diabetes, arthritis, high blood pressure and other degenerative conditions. They played a little bit each day. They got stronger and felt better. One woman, after using crutches for three years, was able to throw them away, stating, "I've put my life in soccer."

Word got out about the soccer grannies. People made fun of them at first. In their traditional roles, these grannies should be at home taking care of their grandkids, cooking, and cleaning. It was unheard of for a grandmother to don shorts and sports shoes. They were ridiculed by friends and neighbors. But they kept playing. A sisterhood grew.

There are now over forty women taking part in the granny soccer league. Other teams formed in neighboring communities. There are regular granny soccer matches. Crowds gather to watch these women strut their stuff. At the end of their game, these ladies will go home and return to cooking, cleaning, and doing what is expected of them. For a moment in time, however, these ladies lose themselves in play. When they finish, they hook arms, sing, and dance off the field. Sisters, all of them.

2 | Create Your Active-Living Vision

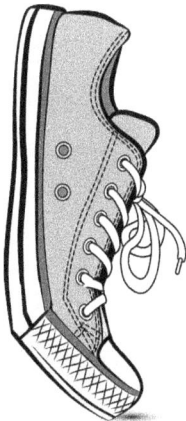

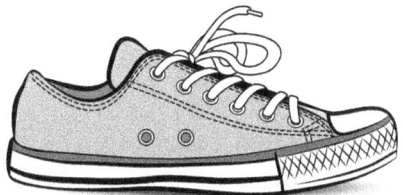

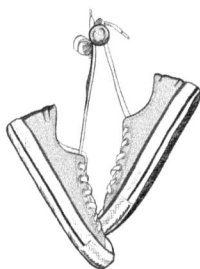

Create Your Active-Living Vision

WHEN TRYING TO CHANGE A behavior, we often jump in and make goals first thing. Although it sounds good, this well-intentioned strategy gets lost because goals need to be tied to a vision, or something bigger than what goals can provide. A vision connects with how you ultimately want to be in the world. It connects you to a better you. Once you settle on your vision or how you see yourself actually living actively, goals serve as stepping stones to guide your path.

Thinking about a vision is a valuable time for reflection. How do you want to be in the world with respect to physical activity and exercise? If you could forget about all the reasons for *not* being active, what would be left? What would living an active life look like for you? Start thinking about how exercise could work for you. Don't let any "yes, but's" enter your mind. What I know for sure is that before outward change can happen, the *thinking* about change from the inside out needs to happen. Start envisioning how you want to live actively.

Who do you want to be? Imagine you are already there; you've lost all the weight and are living actively every day, for example. Describe the active life you see for yourself. Fantasize in the present. Paint a picture of what you do each day. Do you walk in the morning? Do you sneak out at your lunch time to find "me time"? Do you see a personal trainer? Are you preparing to run or walk a 5K? Do you belong to a ballroom dance club? How about stand-up paddle boarding? Do you meet friends in a group exercise class? How does it feel to be active? The possibilities are endless. This is a great time of discovering what you want for yourself.

> In order to carry a positive action, we must develop here a positive vision.
> — *Dalai Lama*

Next, think about your past experiences. Have you been active in years past? What activities did you do? What did you like about those activities? Were they fun? What made you successful? How did you feel? What made you successful with exercise? How did your environment support your success? Did you plan ahead? Did you have active friends? What strengths did you use that you can draw upon now? If you were never active in the past, think about successful times that made you feel good about yourself. What were the specifics about the situation that you liked? What strengths did you rely on? What we are doing here is looking at our past with the eyes of appreciation. What good do you see in your past that you can use today as you move forward?

An active-living vision is most effective if it focuses is on what you want as opposed to what you don't want. Instead of saying, "I want to stop lying on the couch after work," suggest to yourself that, "I want to walk for 15 minutes after work." Set up positive vibes for yourself. Take time to develop your vision. Think about it during the day and let ideas resonate with you. You don't have to write it down all at once. You can start with a brainstorming type of approach. Write down a few things that resonate with you, think about them for a few days and see what sticks. One thing to remember with regard to your active-living vision is that it is not set in stone. Feel free to change it as you grow and learn about what works for you. You also may grow into and out of various physical activities; for example, you might begin a walking program and progress to running—or vice versa if you realize that running just isn't for you.

Here are examples of visions for living an active life:

- I am living a health active life playing tennis regularly and through my healthy choices I am able to control my weight, blood pressure, and stress levels.
- I wake up every morning with a peaceful feeling and ready to embrace the day. I have an active life of walking, yoga and class activities as a natural part of my lifestyle.
- I am living a balanced life. I have an invigorating business and a personal life full of family and friends. I live an active lifestyle of regular exercise. I ride my road bike regularly. I have a daily meditation practice which feeds my spirit.

- I walk every day.

There is no right way to state a vision to live actively. Write what feels best for you.

Be Clear on Why it is Important to You

Why do you want to get active? What is motivating you to change? We know that behavior change is more likely to be successful when we identify with why we want to change. Why does getting active matter to you right now? You can go to the "Pre-Contemplation" (page 38) worksheet to help with this. These questions provide the groundwork for success. Your answers get you thinking and believing that an active life can be yours. They will also be there when you need a pick-me-up moment or a time for reflection to strengthen your resolve. According to Wellcoaches, your vision is "the key that unlocks the door to self-efficacy and self-esteem when it comes to health, fitness and wellness."[3] Your answers to these questions are your new BFF! They will be there for you when the going gets tough.

The following are questions to help define your vision and how to navigate the journey to living an active life.

What do you value?

Values are the things you believe are important in the way you live and work. What you value determines priorities. Look back on situations that made you feel proud, happy, and most fulfilled. These may or may not have anything to do with physical activity. What do you value about these situations? Why do you like doing certain things? What you value helps provide parameters with which to make choices which move you toward an active life. These are the things that are important to you. Do you value being outside with nature? Do you value variety? Do you value alone time? Do you love being with girlfriends? A friend of mine, Kim, began walking regularly with some friends. Here are her comments about what it has meant for her:

> For me, being accountable to two other people gets me out of bed, excited to see them both and share our stresses and delights!!! The energy generated is addicting and I can't imagine a morning without our walk/hike through our town!

When you align what you appreciate and value with your activity, it helps define what kinds of activities you might find enjoyable so that the experience becomes about more than just exercise.

Knowledge is Power

One of the most powerful things you can do when learning to change a health behavior is to learn about the change you want to make. There is a myriad of misinformation circulating around about what is the best kind of exercise, the best type of equipment, the best way to strengthen the core—the list is endless. How do you know if a source of information is based on evidence? The resources at the end of this book are a good place to start. What I like about these sites is that the information is reliable and factual, and it is evidence based.

What about other health/fitness websites, articles, books and advertisements? Research the background of the person providing the information. Do they have a degree in their area of expertise? What are their certifications? What kind of experience do they have? Who endorses them? The health and fitness industry is filled with unqualified experts touting various methods to get fit, so be aware and informed, and when in doubt, ask a qualified health care provider.

Health Coaching

The explosion of the health and wellness coaching industry may be the missing link in our fractured healthcare system. According to the International Consortium for Health and Wellness Coaching (ICHWC), "health and wellness coaches partner with clients seeking self-directed, lasting changes, aligned with their values, which promote health and wellness and, thereby, enhance well-being." The key words, at least to me, are "lasting change." You are the expert in your life and a health coach helps you discover your answers.

The formation of the ICHWC began in 2010 when thought leaders in the field realized that, because of the numerous health coaching programs, a set of national standards was needed to define the field and protect the public. Representatives from nearly 70 health coaching programs, over several years' time, ultimately defined the foundational background of a health coach, the definition of the role, tasks and competencies, scope of practice, code of ethics and how coaching is differentiated from other allied health professions.

Another exciting development is the partnering of ICHWC and the National Board of Medical Examiners (NBME). The NBME, founded in

1915, is an independent, not-for-profit organization that serves the public through its high-quality assessments of healthcare professionals. Together, the ICHWC and the NBME launched the first national board certification for health and wellness coaches in 2017. Over 1100 coaches sat for and passed the exam. When you hire a National Board Certified Health and Wellness Coach, you are hiring a professional who has demonstrated a standard skill level at applying evidence-based practices to assist in achieving your health and wellness goals.

To find a National Board Certified Health and Wellness Coach, go to: https://ichwc.org/directory/

> *Knowledge is power. Information is liberating. Education is the premise of progress, in every society, in every family.*
> —Kofi Annan

Gain Perspective

Take a step back from your active-living vision and think about where you are right now and where you ultimately want to be. Don't forget to give yourself credit for the little things you may already be doing right now. For example, maybe you are parking farther away from the grocery store. Or maybe you are walking fifteen minutes at your lunch hour. Often overlooked, these small active steps foster a sense of self efficacy, which in turn, creates a path for future success. When you look at what you are doing now and what you ultimately want to be able to do, how big is the space between the two? Be objective and accept where you are now. Show yourself some love! Forward movement is hindered when you cannot accept where you are in the present. It might help to detail where you are now on paper under column A. List how you live each day currently. In column B, list how you want to live in your active-living vision. Be honest with yourself. It may be very clear that a big gap exists between the two. No worries! This book will arm you with the tools and insight you need to gradually change into your better self.

How Confident Do You Feel?

How confident you are about being able to close the space between a sedentary life to one of activity? On a scale of 0-10, with 10 being very confident and 0 being not at all confident, how confident are you that you can close this gap? Generally, an answer of 7 and above indicates readiness to change. If you answer less than 7, it might help to rethink how you want to proceed. There is no right or wrong answer other than being honest about your feelings toward change. How ready do you feel to start living actively?

> *We gain strength, and courage, and confidence by each experience in which we really stop to look fear in the face... we must do that which we think we cannot.*
>
> —Eleanor Roosevelt

What are your challenges?

When I owned my health and fitness education business, I used to teach a class called Environmental Control in which I talked about the power the environment has on choices we make. What are situations that you feel will make it difficult to stay on your new track to change? Is it the work environment or your home environment? Do you feel short on time, as though there are not enough hours in a day to fit it all in? Do you foresee potential challenges?

You can learn to plan ahead for these difficult situations. The goal is not to get rid of the situations but to learn how to handle them with a conscious approach, keeping your active-living vision in your forethought. What are some resources, people, or environments that can serve to support you

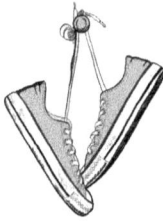

Stories That Inspire Us

ABBY HAD A VERY BUSY social life. She raised four kids who were now grown. She had been the cheerleader for her kids as well as for her husband, who was a physician.

Abby was in the habit of using her social events as reasons to get in shape and lose weight. With a social engagement on the calendar, a few months prior to the date, Abby would hire a personal trainer and go on restrictive diets. After the social event passed, Abby would return to her normal life of inactivity and overeating.

This pattern went on for several years. As each social engagement approached, she felt deprived, tired, and angry. She stated that she often felt resentful of her trainer for taking her through a high-intensity workout. In addition, she was in the habit of allowing other things (be they trainers or diets) to dictate her actions.

When describing her active-living vision, she stated that she was tired of feeling like a yo-yo and not having choices. What she failed to realize is that she did have choices and she chose to be dictated to.

Abby learned, over time, to think about what she wanted without letting herself being dictated to; she finally asked herself the question, "What do I want for myself?" She stopped taking advice from others and gradually incorporated a walking program and yoga into her everyday life.

She worked with a personal trainer occasionally to fine-tune her program. She aligned what she did with what she valued on the inside.

Now when social events occur, Abby no longer stresses out, and looks forward to them without feeling deprived or resentful.

Worksheet:
My Active-Living Vision

This vision is a statement about who you are and what you want to do consistently to support your best active self. The following are some questions to help you in the process of coming to your own mission statement.

- The things I want to do to be active are:

- The reasons I want to be active are:

- The things that I really value and want to incorporate into my life are:

- My past positive experiences with being active include:

- My challenges to living an active life include:

- I plan to use the following support systems when I am feeling overwhelmed, tired, and unfocused:

- My strengths that I can draw upon to overcome these challenges include:

- I will use the following tactics when I find myself feeling impatient:

- On a scale of 1 to 10 with 10 being extremely confident, I feel _____ confident in being able to realize my active-living vision.

- What would make my vision one number higher on the scale?

in your desire to change and become more active?
Start identifying your support systems.

Sarah is someone I worked with a few years ago.
Her story is an example of learning to adapt to a
difficult situation. She had been actively involved
in planning her meals for the week, keeping a food
journal and walking regularly. She then had to go
on a family trip. Her trip proved difficult to stay
on track with her food choices and exercise; her
traditional approach would have been to throw all
she had worked for out the window and eat whatever she wanted, sleep in, and forget exercise. She
came back feeling very positive instead, because
she applied the notion of living in the grey area
of life. She simply remained conscious of choices;
so although she didn't eat as healthy as she did at
home, she stayed away from bread and other car-
bohydrate foods. And she walked every day—even
if it was only twenty minutes. Success!

Helpful Thoughts:

❯ I will not try to be perfect.
❯ I will do the best I can in each situation.
❯ I will remember the phrase "progress, not
perfection."

This may seem complicated at first, but it does get easier! Remember: patience, planning ahead, and a willingness to feel a bit uneasy at times. This is normal! Try not to fret, and take each day one at a time.

> *If there is no struggle, there is no progress.*
> — Federick Douglass

Patience: Your New Friend

This is one of the hardest parts about behavior change. When we want something, we want it *now*. What happens is that we start a vigorous exercise program using the "all or nothing" approach. It feels better to be *doing* something rather than thinking about how to be successful. This approach does not work. Take a look at gym attendance in the month of January compared to March. Gyms sell memberships with the understanding that only 18% of new members will actually use them. When you find yourself feeling impatient or frustrated with slow results, the following tips may help:

Helpful Thoughts:

❯ Become aware of your impatient thoughts. This helps create space from your monkey mind (a

Buddhist term meaning unsettled). Doing this can help separate you from your thoughts and remember the process.

> Take a deep breath. Inhale through your nose, letting in a positive thought. Exhale through your mouth, letting the "bad vibe" thoughts leave. Remember your commitment to why learning to live an active life is important to you.

> Create a rescue message for yourself. Something like, "I can do this and I am worth it."

> Pat yourself on the back for having the awareness to notice your impatience.

Patience is not simply the ability to wait—
it's how we behave while we're waiting.
—Joyce Meyer

3 | Stages of
Change

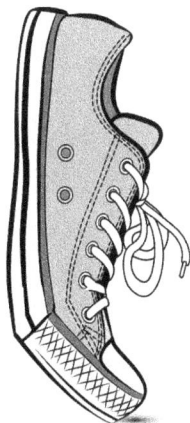

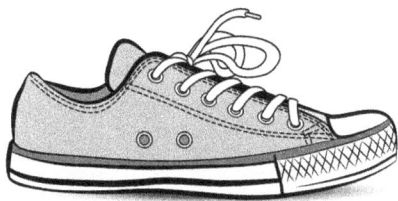

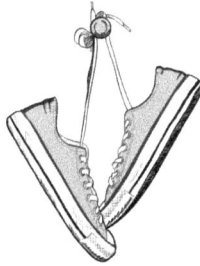

Stages of Change: Your Key to Success

UNDERSTANDING HOW WE CHANGE CREATES a perspective and allows all the "should" thinking to fade away. When readiness to move forward is illuminated, one feels understanding and acceptance.

What I have seen as typical behavior is this scenario: someone wants to lose weight, so they think, "Go out and exercise. Hard! Fast! Every day! Gung ho!" I call this the epic fail setup alert. This action-oriented intervention presumes the way to succeed is a simple matter of stop and go. The reality is that behavior change, in fact, doesn't happen all at once. It is a gradual process which can offer insight into how we think and feel. The big benefit is learning what works for us. And while we want to go from A to Z, what is really needed is to go from A to B. Get to know who you are, what you want, why you want it, and how to do it from the inside out.

This effective model of behavior change was developed by Dr. James Prochaska. According to Wellcoaches, this model "is a blueprint for effecting self-change in health behaviors," including exercise. Here are descriptions of change stages. As you read through them, consider where you might find yourself in these descriptions.

STAGE 1
Not Considering or Not Interested: Pre-Contemplation

I call this the "Not Even Close to Thinking About It" stage: If you are not interested in starting an exercise program, I wonder, then, why are you reading this book? Perhaps you've got just a tickle of an idea to get active? People at this stage fall into two types of thought: those who think, "I won't," and those who think, "I can't." There is nothing wrong in thinking, "I will not exercise." Your doctor, loved one or wellness coach cannot make you move.

I had a client, Jane, who was referred to me by her doctor. She hated exercise, yet her doctor told her she had to move. Jane was so defensive about not wanting to exercise that her defensiveness was keeping her from even thinking of the *possibility* of getting active. There was no room in her thinking, and there was nothing I could do or say. What I did end up doing was acknowledging her feelings about exercise. I told her to contact me if she ever decided that she was ready for activity.

In my experience, people get so tired of being told to exercise that a defense mechanism type of thinking begins to take hold and prevent even the thought of trying to do something. Defensive thinking does not allow for a different approach. How defensive are you about exercise? Are you willing to look at getting active in a different way? One thing you can do at this stage is to simply think about what it would feel like to be more active. Maybe each morning before you get up, think about what living an active life would feel like.

On the other hand, if you find yourself thinking, "I can't exercise," perhaps you have tried and failed in the past. You may have anxiety around physical activity. This is common, and you are certainly not the only person who feels nervous when thinking about starting to get active. Maybe you know you need to start being more active but cannot see a way to be successful. You might be so focused on the reasons and conditions why you can't, that you are unable to see a way out. Realizing the positive reasons to exercise can be helpful in taking the next step.

STAGE 2
Contemplation, or, "I May Get Active"

I call this the "Starting to Think About Maybe Doing Something" stage: If you are thinking about the possibility of becoming more active, you are in a great place! You are beginning to see the costs of an inactive life vs. benefits of living actively. And you are beginning to think that maybe, just maybe, you could see what all the fuss is about. Ultimately, your positive reasons to change must outweigh reasons to stay the same. Many people remain at this stage for years without moving forward. They cannot imagine themselves living an active life, or they don't know where to begin. I do believe, however, in learning about the change process, you gain perspective and are better able to navigate forward movement. In creating your Active-Living Vision Worksheet, you were prompted to explore past experiences as well as reasons to get active in the future. Gain a hopeful perspective in detailing your reasons to get active and how living an active life will feel.

Think back to your Active-Living Vision. You were asked about values—those internal motivators that are important to you. These motivators help form a strong base for forward movement. Listen to other people's stories about how they became more active. Weight Watchers celebrity spokesperson Jennifer Hudson states in her approach to activity that, "…moving is better than doing nothing." With an 80-pound weight loss under her belt, she is a grand example of simply moving more.

> *Every day I'm thinking about change.*
> —Miuccia Prada

STAGE 3
Preparation "I Will"

This is the "I'm Going To Do This" stage. If you plan to get active in the near future, you are feeling more confident about moving forward. You have addressed the cognitive part, or the "thinking, and learning goals" on getting active (more on this later). Such goals might include tasks like gathering information, i.e., reading articles/books on exercise, watching documentaries relating to health/ fitness, and observing fitness classes. You may set a small activity goal of a ten minute daily walk. All of these tasks can help to increase knowledge, decrease anxiety, and boost confidence of success. The more thought that goes into preparing and and strategizing, the better your brain will respond. New neural pathways can develop to support new possibilities. Take a moment to write down a formal statement of what you want to achieve. Then devise small steps you can take each week.

> *Before anything else, preparation is the key to success.* —Alexander Graham Bell

STAGE 4
I Am Active: Action!

In this "Action" stage, you are clear on why you want to get active; you have invested time and energy into learning about activity and its benefits and why it is important to you. Activities have been identified that will work for you; for example, beginning a walking program. You are clear on strategies to have in place to realize success. Now it is time to put the plan into practice. The goal at this stage is to remain conscious of your efforts to stay active. You may spend up to six months in this stage. Lapses and relapses are normal. Setbacks are a positive opportunity to learn what works and doesn't work. Remember, there is no failure—only learning about what will work better next time!

Action is the foundational key to all success.
— Pablo Picasso

A key factor for success at this stage is to remain conscious about the steps being taken in your new active life. The planning part is still important at this stage. Continue to be aware of your thought patterns; don't let the old negative thoughts run the new positive thoughts out of the playing field. Continue to plan ahead for difficult situations and how they may sabotage your best efforts.

STAGE 5
I Am Still Active!

Being successful with any health behavior (including exercise) for six months will put you in this maintenance stage. Confidence is strong, and you are feeling a new sense of self-efficacy through regular exercise. You've done a great job! Prevent boredom by creating new challenges. Perhaps you might be ready to work toward meeting the American College of Sports Medicine's definition of cardiovascular exercise, which suggests that exercise be done 3-5 times a week for 20-60 minutes at a moderate to high level of intensity. Or, if you are already at that level, perhaps adding a new activity or running a 5K? Challenges at this stage are fun! See where your newfound fitness can take you.

> *I've learned in my life that it's important to be able to step outside your comfort zone and be challenged with something you're not familiar or accustomed to. That challenge will allow you to see what you can do.* —J.R. Martinez

One thing that happens when people realize success is that they continue doing the same thing because that is what worked for them. There is really nothing wrong with this approach unless you begin to feel bored. Look at boredom as an opportunity to try something new. For example, you can up the intensity of your walk to include small bouts of jogging; you can start to do some hills in your neighborhood; you can finally try out that Zumba class that your girlfriends rave about. The opportunities are endless. Just try one thing and see what happens. Variety is the spice of life, especially when it comes to physical activity. Many of my clients remark that when they vary their day-to-day routine, the time goes faster and before they realize it, the week has passed with every day filled with some sort of activity. So don't be afraid to experiment.

Where do you see yourself in these stages?

Do you want to move forward regardless of the stage where you find yourself? Forward movement is possible when the process of change is clear. You might feel like a failure for starting and stopping regular exercise so many times. You are not alone. To realize success, goals need to meet you at your stage of change. So perhaps when you "failed" in the past, you simply did not match intended goals with where you find yourself. Try to move away from the black and white approach to exercise. Your active-living vision, your stage of change, and your goals are created in the grey area of life—a fluid state of internal mindfulness. This is where the mystery happens. Read further to begin your transformation to joy through physical activity.

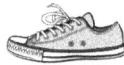

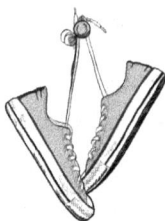

Stories That Inspire Us

THE BOOK SECRET STAIRS: *A Guide to the Historic Staircases of Los Angeles* by Charles Fleming, is a spanking great read about little-known urban adventures just waiting to be discovered. Fleming spent hours studying, measuring, mapping and photographing the hidden stairways of Los Angeles. As a mini history lesson, a walk among these hidden stairways gives a glimpse into a more innocent time when people walked more than drove. The stairs helped navigate the endless hills of the City of Angels.

The book is divided up into five sections, each representing a particular area of Los Angeles. Each section has between four and eleven various walks that are measured in the number of stairs, the length of walk and the measure of difficulty. These walks are a treasure map to enchantment.

But here is what I really like about this book.

Before discovering these staircases, Fleming was a broken man. He had undergone two hip surgeries and a hand surgery and he had suffered a broken leg. He had also endured two spinal surgeries. He was still in constant pain. His doctor recommended yet a third surgery. He declined.

Then he tried something different. He started walking. At first he walked a modest two blocks—about as much as he could tolerate. After doing this for a period of time, he found his pain became more tolerable. It was during these early walks that he discovered the first stairs in the Silver Lake area of Los Angeles. As he began to feel better, he worked up to half a mile. And then another. He ended up searching for and discovering a trove of hidden gems throughout the city. He became stronger. And he never had that third back surgery.

To me, the lesson serves as a reminder that physical activity can be an answer to your prayers. Walking can take you away from something crummy toward something better. Perhaps there are some hidden staircases in your neck of the woods?

Worksheet
Stage 1: Pre Contemplation

Raise Your Pros!
A "Not Even Close to Thinking About It" Activity

Help yourself become friendly with the wondrous benefits of physical activity. Below are reasons to get moving. Which reasons feel good for you? Check off those that spark your interest. The more reasons you have to begin, the easier it will be to get moving. Enjoy this exercise.

Physical Health
❏ Helps manage weight
❏ Helps lose weight (with calorie reduction)
❏ Helps improve heart lung and muscle fitness
❏ Helps to raise "good" HDL cholesterol
❏ Helps to decrease risk of clogged blood vessels
❏ Helps lower resting heart rate
❏ Helps to decrease irregular heart rhythms
❏ Helps improve circulation
❏ Helps to improve immune function
❏ Helps immune system work better
❏ Helps the body use insulin better
❏ Helps to strengthens joints
❏ Helps to strengthens bones
❏ Helps improves cardiovascular function

❑ Helps to decrease risk of many illnesses, including diabetes, depression and stroke and heart disease

❑ Helps to improve balance

❑ Helps to improve posture

Intellectual Health

❑ You will feel less nervous or anxious

❑ You will feel more alert

❑ You will improve your memory

❑ You will experience decreased depressive thoughts

❑ You will better able to handle stress

❑ You will feel less anger

❑ You will be easier to be around

❑ You will experience less tension headaches

❑ You will feel less muscle tension

Emotional Health

❑ You will feel better about yourself

❑ You will like yourself more

❑ You will like others more

❑ You will begin to see possibilities

❑ You will learn how to tap into who you are inside

❑ You will learn what works and doesn't work for you

❏ You feel better about saying "no"
❏ You will no longer worry about what others
   think
❏ You will be easier to be around
❏ You will have a more positive outlook on life
❏ You will feel successful!

Now it's your turn. Think of reasons to get active
versus reasons to stay sedentary.

REASONS TO...	
GET ACTIVE	**STAY THE SAME**
1.	1.
2.	2.
3.	3.
4.	4.
5.	5.

Which list is longest? Your answer will give an
idea of how ready you are to change.

Worksheet
Stage 2: Contemplation

"I May Get Active"
Overcome Your Barriers!
A "Starting to Think About
Maybe Doing Something" Activity

Complete the "Raise Your Pros" activity. Becoming more aware of what your "pros" to activity are will help overcome your barriers.

YOUR TOP 5 BARRIERS TO EXERCISE	YOUR TOP 5 SOLUTIONS
Example: I don't have time	I can walk for 15 minutes during my lunch hour on Monday, Wednesday and Friday
1.	1.
2.	2.

YOUR TOP 5 BARRIERS TO EXERCISE	YOUR TOP 5 SOLUTIONS
3.	3.
4.	4.
5.	5.

One helpful thought to keep in mind is that many little bits of activity add up to a lot. If you can't figure out how to walk for forty-five minutes, try adding little bits during the day. This tip can apply to activities other than walking, too.

Prepare to Move!
An "I Am Going to Do This" Activity

My Action Plan
Start Date:
Days of the week I will exercise:

	Time of Day	Activity	Location	Time	Backup Plan
MON					
TUE					
WED					
THU					
FRI					
SAT					
SUN					

- Things I need to do to get started (i.e., check out local gyms, choose a class, map out walking route, etc.):

- What I need to buy before starting (i.e., shoes, activity monitor, hat, mP3 player, etc.):

- Other steps I can take to prepare: (schedule babysitter, plan meals for dinner, pack my lunch for work):

Helpful Thoughts:

> If I find myself feeling too tired, I will remember how much more energy I will have after I exercise.
> If I am feeling too stressed out to exercise, I will look at my exercise time as a mental vacation.
> If I am feeling too busy to exercise, I will remember my new way of thinking of exercise as a vital part of a healthy and busy life.

Stage 4: I Am Active

Action!
I am Doing This Activity!

Conscious Actions

	Conscious Action Examples:
MORNING	Get up 20 minutes early and go for a walk and have my clothes where they are easy to put on; go to the gym before work, pack my gym bag the night before.
NOONTIME	Go for a 20-minute walk at my lunch hour, which still leaves me time to eat my pre-planned healthy lunch; take a noontime fitness class with my already-packed gym bag ready to go; start a walking club at work.
EVENING	Go to the gym before I get home from work; go for a walk at a park on my way home from work; go for a bike ride with my neighbor after work; go to a yoga class on my way home from work.

	Conscious Action Examples:
WEEKENDS	Participate in family activities like going for a hike or a bike ride; join a singles hiking group for weekend hikes.
SOCIAL SITUATIONS	Plan ahead by eating before going to a party; drink plenty of water during the event; bring healthy food choices to a potluck event; make sure I get my walk in before going to the event.

- Now it is your turn. List the potential times you can fit any sort of activity into your life, along with any situations that may present challenges to your intended goals.

- How does exercise help you reach your goals?

- What unexpected situations can get you off track?

- How will you handle them?

	Conscious Action Examples:
MORNING	
NOONTIME	

	Conscious Action Examples:
EVENING	
WEEKENDS	
SOCIAL SITUATIONS	

Worksheet

Stage 5: I Am Still Active

Maintenance Stage
An "I Am Still Doing This!" Activity

- My top three physical activities:

- On a typical day, here is how I feel before my workout:

- On a typical day, here is how I feel during my workout:

- On a typical day, here is how I feel after my workout:

- What can I do, if anything, to help me stay motivated to continue with my plan?

- What are some activities that I want to try?

- What are some upcoming events that I would like to participate in?

- How can I best prepare for these events?

Things No One Tells You

Get Comfortable With Being Uncomfortable

Discomfort can come in the form of physical exertion, or it can come in the form of mental anxiety. When changing any behavior, a certain level of disquiet is experienced. Acknowledge that this is normal and that it is okay to feel this feeling. You will learn to move through that feeling and get to a new level of being. This is where I see many get stuck. Some level of discomfort must be felt in order to move forward. So when asking how ready you are to change, also ask yourself if you are willing to push through that icky feeling of discomfort, be it physical or emotional.

> *Move out of your comfort zone. You can only grow if you are willing to feel awkward and uncomfortable when you try something new.*
> —Brian Tracy

Setbacks

This is another one of those "icky" things no one wants to feel when trying to change.

Relapse can happen at any time during the change process. It happens to everybody, no matter what level of fitness. Injury, illness, a new baby or job all can have an impact on activity levels. Here is what to remember: there is no shame. It happens to all of us. Look at this awful feeling as an opportunity to learn what works and doesn't work for you. Take an objective look at what the triggers were for relapse. Create some space between you and your behavior. You are not what you do. Acknowledge the barriers and create steps to overcome them next time. Go to your active-living vision worksheet and reaffirm what you want for yourself and your reasons to get active. Re-evaluate, readjust, and show yourself some love. Salute positive successes. If your setback is due to injury, remember that the injury doesn't have to prevent you from living actively. Start back slowly and ask your healthcare provider the best way to proceed. With mindful thought, relapse stages become shorter and less frequent. They will no longer have the power to derail your intentions. That is success!

> *Rather than viewing a brief relapse back to inactivity as a failure, treat it as a challenge and try to get back on track as soon as possible.* —Jimmy Connors

Worksheet:
Tips for the Discouraged or Impatient Thinkers

- Take a deep breath. This helps create perspective.
- Recognize your successes so far. This helps build a sense of separation from where you began and a sense of realizing that you are doing more than you had been doing.
- Remember that it takes a long time to change. This is normal! Show yourself some love and accept yourself for your efforts thus far.
- Go for a walk! Even a fifteen minute walk can help break negative thought patterns.
- Remember that there is always more than one way to look at a situation—a positive way and a negative way. You have control over which one you choose.
- Give yourself a chance to get over the humps and bumps along the way toward your more active life. Change is never a straight shot!
- Remember, anything you do is better than nothing at all.
- Call a friend.
- Volunteer for an organization you feel strongly about. One of the best ways to change how we feel about ourselves is to give to others.

- Clean house. I know that sounds ridiculous, but many of my clients have stated that it gets their mind off of things, gets them moving and allows them to feel a sense of accomplishment. One client remarked that she puts on her favorite music with her headphones and goes into "la-la land." (Her words, not mine!) This is a great example of finding what works for YOU.

Write down three things you can do when feeling discouraged or impatient:

1.

2.

3.

> *You can't change who you are, but you can change what you have in your head, you can refresh what you're thinking about, you can put some fresh air in your brain.* —Ernesto Bertarelli

4 | Goal Setting

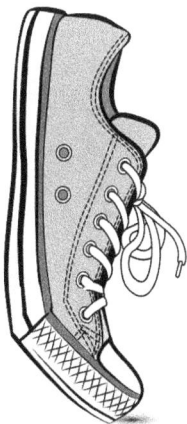

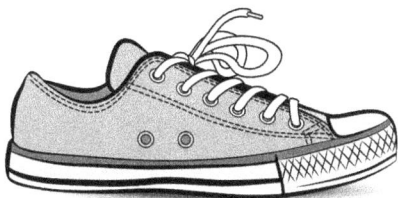

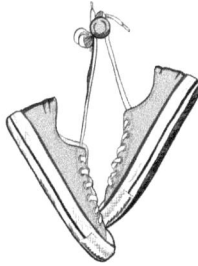

Goal Setting: Your Ticket to Success

Setting goals is the first step in turning the invisible into the visible.— Tony Robbins

NOW THAT YOU HAVE YOUR vision about how you want to be, it's time to bring back into the picture the concept of goal setting. This is an opportunity to use your creativity and have some fun! I like to call this process "Self-design your path to success." Goals should be created from a space of optimism and positive energy. You don't have to—you *get* to! Goals are your building blocks to success and can be your new BFF.

Here is the thing about goals: not only will they provide structure to the change process, they help develop a sense of self-efficacy, an important and often overlooked feeling when it comes to behavior change. Self-efficacy is the belief that you can be successful. As success builds upon itself, setting appropriate goals helps foster success and thus self-efficacy. There are two types of goals whose use is determined by where you are in the change process. Look back at how you answered Worksheets 1 and 2.

Thinking/Feeling/Learning Goals

If you find yourself in the earlier stage of change, congratulations on recognizing where you are right now. You have a wonderful opportunity to learn new things! These types of goals are often referred to by behavior change experts as the "gathering of information" goals. You can start to learn about yourself and what interests you. You can talk to people who have learned to live actively. What worked for them? Seek out support from others. Remember, remain open and teachable. Be aware of any mind games that want to tear you down.

These cognitive goals are used in the contemplation and preparation stages. How can you increase your awareness of getting more active? Noticing headlines in the paper, reading books, watching documentaries, getting pamphlets from your doctor's office all are ways to start a new way of thinking about living actively. Become aware of your feelings when reading about exercise. Make note of certain social trends—signs encouraging taking the stairs instead of the elevator, for example. Have new walking paths opened up near your office or home? What are some ways you can work out at home, such as fitness DVDs or Wii Sports activities. Notice your effect on others, too. How do you interact with your family or coworkers when you don't exercise? How can you set an example for your children?

These are just a few examples of how you can begin the process of *thinking* more actively. The list is endless, too. Can you create a top five list of things to do over the next month? Use this as an opportunity for self-care.

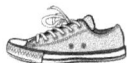

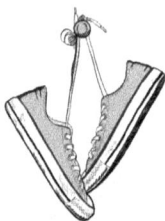

Stories That Inspire Us

CARMINE HAD A HISTORY OF starting an exercise program only to stop after a few short months.

She would start gung ho with whatever craze was popular at the time, partaking in the activity 5-6 days per week. Yet she somehow felt like it was just too much work to keep it up and stopped.

After years of this approach, Carmine wasn't sleeping well at night, she had gained weight over the years, she was experiencing knee pain, and she just felt as though she would never be a regular exerciser.

When I asked about what made her start these programs, she reiterated that she just wanted to feel better about herself. She was tired of feeling inadequate. She was tired of not fitting into her clothes, too.

In describing her active-living vision, Carmine stated that she just wanted to be able to go to Disneyland and not be wiped out from walking all day. She wanted to take part in activities with her family and friends. She wanted to feel good about herself when she woke up in the morning.

Carmine was suffering from a common misperception: she believed that exercise had to be hard and uncomfortable. Carmine had to change her approach.

Instead of going gung ho and feeling miserable, she had to learn how to develop goals that met where she was. If she wanted to ultimately walk every day for thirty minutes, she first had to get a good pair of shoes, research walking paths in her community, and find some books to listen to on her MP3 player.

These three tasks became her goals starting out. She then had to figure out what time of day would work best for her as well as what days of the week would work best.

Over time, Carmine became a regular walker; she realized that she just didn't want a high intensity program. She took a small, step by step approach and became successful at incorporating a regular walking program into her daily routine.

You too can learn how to break down the big picture into small, manageable steps to feel successful and ultimately move you forward to your vision.

Worksheet:
Early Stage Goals

(Thinking/Feeling Goals)
Acquiring Information—Let's Learn!

Examples of these types of goals all serve to increase your awareness of changes you want to make.

Make a list of activities you can start doing now to get warmed up to the idea of physical activity:

1.

2.

3.

4.

5.

6.

7.

8.

Here are some examples:

1. Checking out my city's online map of walking paths.
2. Reading my local recreation department catalog list of exercise classes.
3. Watching a documentary about the food industry and how it affects our perceptions (refer to resource page for suggestions).
4. Reading about other people who have learned how to live an active life.
5. Noticing how I relate to others when I don't feel so good about myself.
6. Buying a magazine on healthy cooking.
7. Taking a free education class offered through my local hospital.
8. Downloading apps to my phone relating to activity and nutrition.

Be creative. And you don't have to come up with these goals at one time. Let the notion sit with you for a few days and see what you come up with.

Action Goals

Action goals, on the other hand, take you from the thinking about change to the "let's get going" stage in your transformation. Be mindful of where you are now and how you ultimately want to live as you stated in your "Active-Living Vision" worksheet. This is where you can set up short-term and long-term goals.

For example, if a long-term goal is to be able to run a 5K, and you currently do no exercise at all, a shorter-term goal can be something like walking for thirty minutes four days per week. Now, you will need to create more goals to meet that short term goal. As an example, you might state that in order to meet the goal of walking for thirty minutes four days per week, "I am going to start by walking for twenty minutes three days per week." Do you see how there is a staircase progression happening? The wider the gap in your active-living vision, the more short-term goals are needed. Use your creativity to see what will work for you. Remember, trial and error is okay! Perfection is not the goal. Learning what works and what doesn't work *for you* is the goal.

Make Your Goals Smart

You have your active-living vision detailed and long- and short-term goals defined. Now is the time to get smart! A goal is a great idea. Getting there can be a circuitous endeavor. Using the smart goal platform will allow a clear, concise, and attainable goal, ensuring forward movement.

The smart goal platform is a way of writing goals that are specific, measurable, attainable, realistic, and time-based. Writing your goals in this manner does require a bit more thought upfront, but it is well worth it in the long run. I have seen many well-intentioned people get sidetracked from goals that got away from them. Be proactive!

Here is an example of a smartly written goal compared to a less specific goal. On Monday, Wednesday and Friday of next week, I will walk the walking path in twenty minutes at my lunch hour. A poorly written goal could be something like, "I will walk during the week". Do you see the difference?

Once the goal is written, consider how to set yourself up for success. What do you need to do to be successful? Do you need to bring your shoes to work? Pack your lunch at home so that you don't go out? Get your bag ready the night before?

Always consider your environment and how to manage it to support your intentions.

A helpful way to look at a smart goal is that it is what you need to do to achieve a longer term goal—say, of weight loss, for example. I have never been a big fan of using weight loss as a goal in and of itself. It just doesn't work. There is nothing wrong with wanting to lose weight, but the focus must be on what you need to DO to lose the weight.

> *When it is obvious that the goals cannot be reached, don't adjust the goals, adjust the action steps.* —Confucius

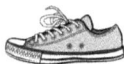

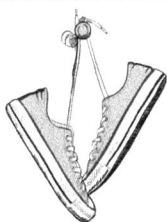

Stories That Inspire Us

CHERYL WORKED IN A MEDICAL office. She had always been active when her kids were young.

As they grew up, however, Cheryl found that her activity levels were not as tied up into playing with her kids. Fast forward to the present.

Cheryl did no exercise when she came to me. Cheryl was able to describe how she wanted to live an active life. She wanted to feel strong again and manage her weight better. She came up with some goals that she felt confident she could meet.

The best time for her to walk was after work. Although at first she was able to meet her goal of walking after work three days per week, it began to be more of a chore after the novelty wore off. She was no longer in the mood to move after a long day of work.

Going back to her active-living vision, she still felt strongly about getting active. We then brainstormed and came up with some ideas she could do instead.

The "a-ha!" moment for Cheryl came when

she realized that anything she did was better than nothing at all, so if she came home from work and rode her stationary bike for fifteen minutes, that was better than nothing.

She kept up with this for a few weeks and then was able to move ahead into her original goal of walking after work—but she started with two days per week at first and the stationary bike at home for a third day.

Feeling successful, she later added a third day of walking, bring her activity level up to four days per week. Cheryl learned how to adjust to her level of comfort, keeping in mind, of course, what her active living vision was.

The point here is that there is a certain amount of fluidity available to you when learning to change what you do—as long as you do something.

Worksheet:
Smart Goals

Smart goals can be tied to thinking or action-based goals. For example, if you are thinking of getting more active in the next six months, here are examples of smart goals that can help you begin thinking actively:

- On Thursday, I will make a list of the five top reasons to get active for next week.
- I will research healthy cooking recipe books on Saturday and make a list of my top three choices.
- On Wednesday at my lunch hour, I will check out a documentary about the food industry at my library and watch it that night.
- On Saturday, I will research books on diet, health, and exercise and choose one to purchase.

Here are five SMART goals that I can start doing right now:

1.

2.

3.

4.

5.

Smart goals can also be action-based. Here are some examples:

- I will walk for twenty minutes during my lunch hour on Tuesday and Thursday.
- I will get up twenty minutes earlier and walk before I have coffee on Monday and Wednesday.
- On Friday, I will walk with my neighbor at 3:00 p.m. for forty-five minutes.

If you are ready for action, make a list of five action goals written using the smart goal platform:

1.

2.

3.

4.

> *What you get by achieving your goals is not as important as what you become by achieving your goals.* —Henry David Thoreau

5 | Mindfulness

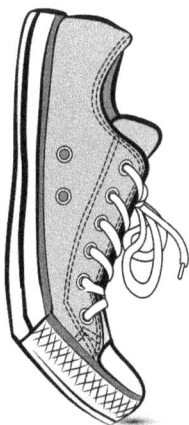

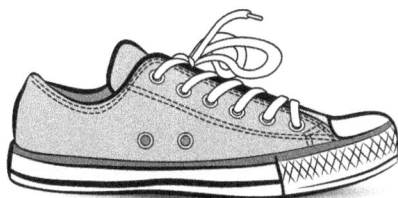

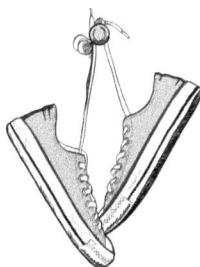

Mindfulness

THE CONCEPT OF MINDFULNESS IS becoming more mainstream; currently, the National Institutes of Health is conducting fifty clinical trials on the subject of mindfulness and health. Mindfulness is a state of attention to the present moment. Being mindful lets you observe your thoughts and feelings without judgment. An important tool for behavior change, mindfulness allows us to experience the present moment without letting thoughts and emotions steer us into the bad choice neighborhood.

In learning to live an active life, being mindful can help tune into the physiological responses to exercise without judgment. So instead of saying, "I hate to sweat," you might begin to re-interpret the feeling of sweating as something good for you. Sweating is really a byproduct of a great self-care activity. It's a good thing. You still may not like the feeling of sweating, but taking a step back and creating space between your thought and the experience helps with perspective. A client, Ann, remarks that as much as she doesn't like the feeling of exertion, she "loves how she feels afterwards." Ann is willing to sweat and breathe hard because she knows that she will better handle whatever comes her way throughout the day. She has learned how to re-frame her mind about sweating.

Contrasting the notion of mindfulness is the tool of distraction. That is, how to distract yourself from looking at the clock while you are working out. If you don't like what you are doing, time crawls by. Tools of distraction can help get over the hump of not liking the feelings of exertion including increased heart rate, body temperature, blood pressure, sweating and possible muscle fatigue. Incorporating tactics such as listening to music, books, podcasts or walking with a friend can help distract from the feeling of exertion.

There is a certain amount of "tuning out" that can occur with distraction, too. Although being able to walk for thirty minutes without it really seeming like thirty minutes is a good thing, being aware of how you feel during that time can sync the feeling of exertion with doing something good for yourself. There is a balance, if you will, of tuning out and tuning in. The notion of mindful walking requires an awareness of the present moment. Being aware of the breath, listening to sounds of nature, traffic, or listening for children playing, noticing the clouds, or noticing people as they pass can help tune into the moment. These are tools for having a nonjudgmental awareness of the present moment. So many times we tend to make choices out of an unrecognized feeling. What would be that choice if we were aware of our underlying emotion? Being comfortable with less-than-perfect conditions is a step in the right direction as you begin to associate physical exertion with a self-care tool in your active living plan.

So which is better—mindfulness or distraction? Having no definitive answer, this question lies in the grey area of life. It is a good conversation to have with yourself when you are learning to live actively. Both play a role in the decision to move forward with physical activity.

Mindfulness Activity

Tuning In vs. Tuning Out

TOOLS OF DISTRACTION EXAMPLES	TOOLS OF MINDFULNESS EXAMPLES
MP3 player	Noticing the environment
Audio books	Noticing the weather
Podcasts	Noticing sounds
Walking with friends	Noticing how I feel
Taking a group exercise class	Noticing my breathing

Now it's your turn.

Here are some ways I can use distraction when I don't feel like exercising:

-

-

-

-

Here are some ways I can tune into myself and learn the art of mindfulness and not judge myself as I learn to become more physically active:

•

•

•

•

Here is another exercise to help bring attention to the present moment: On my walk today, here is what I noticed:

During my drive to work today, I noticed the following:

While on my lunch hour, I took a five-minute break to focus on my breathing. Here is what I felt:

When I got home from work and did not want to go for a walk, here is how I did it anyway:

Mindfulness

6 | Activity Style Assessment

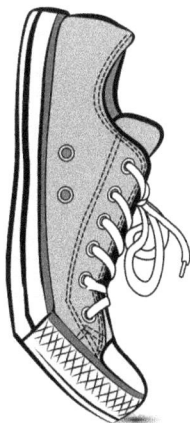

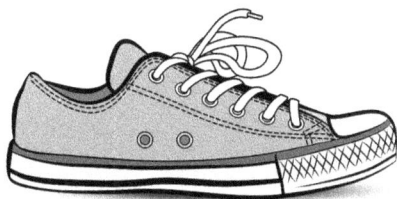

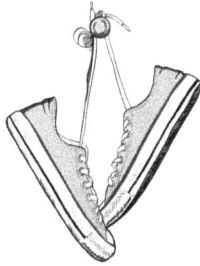

Activity Style
Assessment

IF YOU FEEL AS THOUGH you don't know how to live an active life, you are not alone. I have had clients remark that they feel overwhelmed with the thought of beginning something new. This is an opportunity to look at physical activity in a whole new way. The following list includes various activities categorized according to characteristics to help narrow your choices. Throughout this book, I have often used walking as an example. According to the National Weight Control Registry, 94% of successful weight loss participants increased their physical activity, with walking being the most utilized activity. Is walking for you? I don't know but what I do know is that it is a great place to start.

THESE ACTIVITIES ARE GROUPED BASED on simple characteristics. They are not grouped according to training adaptations such as cardiovascular endurance, muscle strength, flexibility or balance activities. Don't worry about the outcome of exercise at this point. Once you feel confident in living actively, then you can fine tune your program and focus on training adaptations.

Simply place an "X" in the column that best describes how you feel about each activity. Do not rate these activities based on what you feel you "should" like or not like; there are no right or wrong answers-only what is right for you. Be honest and know that there is a way for you to live an active life even if you have never been physically active in the past.

When you are done, the "Willing to Try" column represent activities that will be the best fit for where you are right now. Keep in mind that as you continue to remain active, your interests can broaden and you may find yourself willing to try activities in the other columns, too. I have had many clients check only one activity in the "Willing to Try" column (in most cases it was walking). And although most of them continued to walk, they branched out to try other activities, too.

Once you determine what activities to begin with, the next step is to plug them into your active living vision and your goal setting steps. For example, what do you need to do to begin a walking program? Can you research walking routes in your neighborhood? Purchase a good pair of shoes? What time day works best? Are there any barriers to be aware of? For example, if you want to walk 15 minutes before work three times per week, how can you set yourself up for success? Many clients state they prepare the night before by putting clothes, shoes and iPod ready near their bed.

This following charts gives you a place to start. If you have other activities not listed, by all means try them out! There is only one way to figure out if they will work. Keep an open mind and always refer back to your active living vision to stay focused.

Activity Style Assessment

LEISURE ACTIVITIES				
Activity	No Way	Don't Think So	Perhaps	Willing To Try
Bocce Ball				
Bowling				
Gardening				
Hiking				
Horseshoes				
Walking				

GROUP/SOCIAL ACTIVITIES				
Activity	No Way	Don't Think So	Perhaps	Willing To Try
Badminton				
Ballroom Dance				
Bicycling				
Boxing				
Circuit Training				
Contra Dance				
Cross Fit				
Fencing				
Frisbee				
Frisbee Golf				

GROUP/SOCIAL ACTIVITIES				
Activity	No Way	Don't Think So	Perhaps	Willing To Try
Golf				
Hiking				
Jazzercise				
Jogging				
Modern Dance				
Pilates				
Running				
Skateboard				
Square Dance				
Stroller Strides				
Walking				
Weight Lifting				
Yoga				
Zumba				

SOLO ACTIVITIES				
Activity	No Way	Don't Think So	Perhaps	Willing To Try
Bicycling				

SOLO ACTIVITIES				
Activity	No Way	Don't Think So	Perhaps	Willing To Try
Dancing at Home With No One Watching				
Elliptical				
Hiking				
Jogging				
Jump Rope				
Running				
Skateboard				
Stationary Bike				
Treadmill				
Walking				
Weight Lifting				

TEAM ACTIVITIES				
Activity	No Way	Don't Think So	Perhaps	Willing To Try
Baseball/ Softball				
Basketball				
Beach Volleyball				
Dodgeball				

TEAM ACTIVITIES

Activity	No Way	Don't Think So	Perhaps	Willing To Try
Field Hockey				
Handball				
Hockey				
Kickball				
Pickle ball				
Racquetball				
Squash				
Table Tennis				
Tennis				
Volleyball				

WATER ACTIVITIES

Activity	No Way	Don't Think So	Perhaps	Willing To Try
Aqua Jogging				
Boogie Board				
Canoeing				
Kayaking				
Stand Up Paddleboard				
Surfing				

WATER ACTIVITIES				
Activity	No Way	Don't Think So	Perhaps	Willing To Try
Swimming				
Synchronized Swimming				
Water Aerobics				
Water Polo				

DANCE ACTIVITIES				
Activity	No Way	Don't Think So	Perhaps	Willing To Try
Ballet				
Ballroom Dance				
Contra Dance				
Dancing at Home With No One Watching				
Jazz Dance				
Modern Dance				
Square Dance				
Jazzercise				
Zumba				

COLD WEATHER ACTIVITIES				
Activity	No Way	Don't Think So	Perhaps	Willing To Try
Cross Country Skiing				
Downhill skiing				
Ice Skating				
Snow Shoeing				

MARTIAL ARTS ACTIVITIES				
Activity	No Way	Don't Think So	Perhaps	Willing To Try
Judo				
Jujitsu				
Karate				
Kickboxing				
Taekwondo				

Is Health Coaching For Me?

My hope for you after reading this book is that it has served, at the very least, to get you thinking about getting active. And with this new active thinking, you begin to see that it is possible to be active regardless of your exercise history. That exercise can literally, change your life.

But even with the best of intentions we sometimes need support. If you hate to exercise, if you doctor has told you to start moving, if you have trouble maintaining an active life and are willing to try a different approach, I can help.

During our coaching sessions, you will learn about your strengths and how to use them in creating an active life that fits who you are. You'll discover how to bring activities into your life that work for you. Coaching sessions focus on your desires so if you want coaching around nutrition, stress, sleep or other areas of wellness, I can help with those, too.

Coaching session are over the phone. You can be in your jammies!

The first thing to do is visit my website (**www. joyofactiveliving.com**) and schedule a free consultation. We'll talk about your whys, your past challenges and where you need help.

I look forward to hearing from you!

7 | Resources

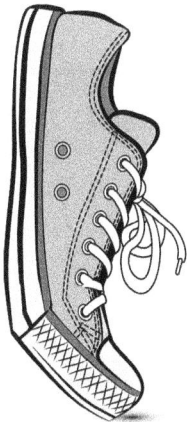

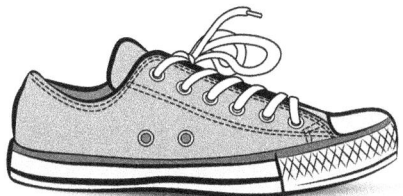

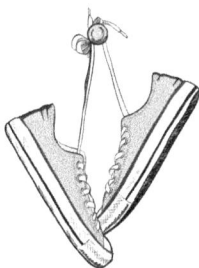

Resources

Organizations

- American College of Sports Medicine
  www.acsm.org

- American Council on Exercise
  www.acefitness.org

- Everybody Walk!   **www.everybodywalk.org**

- Exercise is Medicine
  www.exerciseismedicine.org

- National Strength and Conditioning
  Association   **www.nsca.com**

- National Academy of Sports Medicine
  www.nasm.org

- International Consortium for Health and
  Wellness Coaching   **www.ichwc.org**

- International Health and Fitness
  Association   **www.ideafit.com**

Online resources
(your tax dollars at work!)

- **www.nlm.nih.gov/medlineplus/
  exerciseandphysicalfitness.html**

- **www.supertracker.usda.gov**

- **www.cdc.gov**

- **www.health.gov**
  This is a resource that serves as a collection of
  health initiatives aimed at keeping our nation
  healthy. Included in this site are the following
  pull-down menus:
  » **Healthy People** establishes science-based
    objectives with national targets and assess-
    ing progress throughout the decade
  » **Health Finder** evidence-based, original
    prevention and wellness topics, health
    resources from 1400 government and non-
    profit organizations and digital tools for sup-
    porting and promoting health.
  » **Dietary Guidelines** a wealth of informa-
    tion concerning everything diet-related.
    Dietary guidelines are published every 5
    years; we are due for a new one in 2015.

There are prepackaged workshops available for community education.

» **Physical Activity Guidelines** these guidelines help you understand the importance of physical activity, know the types and amounts of physical activity you need for health, choose the appropriate physical activities that fit into any lifestyle or routine, help others be more physically active, and learn ways to reduce the risks of activity-related injury.

» **Health Literacy and Communication** tools for health professionals to help make health information understandable.

» **Health Care Quality and Patient Safety** learn to be your best advocate in the medical setting. Resources for caregivers and patient safety.

Apps

The following are fitness apps as well as online tools that you can incorporate into everyday life. They each have something to offer and they play an important role in motivation. Check them out to see if they can work for you.

• **www.fitbit.com**

• **www.myfitnesspal.com**

- **www.sparkpeople.com**

Educational Documentaries

- *Escape Fire (2012)*
- *Fat, Sick and Nearly Dead* (2010)
- *Fed Up* (2014)
- *Food, Inc.* (2008)
- *Forks Over Knives* (2011)
- *Supersize Me* (2004)

Books

These books are by no means an exhaustive list. They represent books that I and/or my clients have found helpful in the journey towards living a more active life:

- Borysenko, J. (2009). *It's Not the End of the World: Developing Resilience in Times of Change.* Carlsbad, CA: Hay House, Inc.

- Borysenko, J.(2014). *The Plant Plus Diet Solution.* Carlsbad: Hay House, Inc.

- Brown, R. (2012). *Daring Greatly: How the Courage to Be Vulnerable Transforms the Way We Live, Love, Parent and Lead.* New York: Gotham Books.

- Fleming, C. (2010). *Secret Stairs: A Walking Guide to the Historic Staircases of Los Angeles*. Santa Monica: Santa Monica Press, LLC.

- Hottinger, G. & Scholtz, M. (2012). *Coach Yourself Thin: 5 Steps to Retrain Your Mind, Reclaim Your Power, and Lose the Weight for Good*. New York: Rodale, Inc.

- Hyman, M. (2014). *10-Day Detox Diet*. New York: Little Brown and Company.

- Levin, N. (2014). *Jump and Your Life Will Appear: An Inch by Inch Guide to Making a Major Change*. Carlsbad, CA: Hay House Inc.

- Moore, M., & Tschannen Moran, B. (2010). *Coaching Psychology Manual*. Philadelphia: Lippincott, Williams and Wilkins.

- Pollan, M. (2009). *Food Rules*. New York: Penguin Books

- Segar, M. (2015). *No Sweat: How the Simple Science of Motivation Can Bring You a Lifetime of Fitness*. New York: AMACOM.

- Wogahn, Melissa, "*How to Get Active and Stay Active: 5 Insights to Shift Your Attitude*." **www.joyofactiveliving.com**

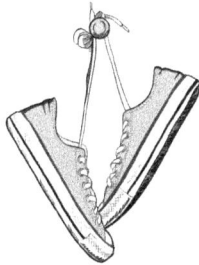

Notes

- 1 **https://www.cdc.gov/nchs/fastats/exercise. htm**

- 2 Bernstein, Lenny. "5 years of fitness reporting and 1 lesson: just move." The Washington *Post*, 4 March, 2014

- 3 Moore, M., & Tschannen Moran, B. (2010). *Coaching Psychology Manual*. Philadelphia: Lippincott, Williams and Wilkins

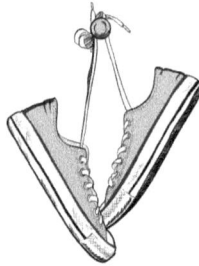

Acknowledgments

One never completes a project like this on their own. I want to thank my publisher for the constant guidance on everything. I could not have completed this project this without your wisdom. Thank you to my editor, Lane, for your valuable and witty suggestions. I would also like to thank the Southern California Wellcoaches Alliance, for offering support, encouragement and meaningful questions in guiding the message *Off The Couch*. I would also like to thank my clients over the years who have demonstrated bravery and tenacity in forging their path forward in living their own active life from the inside out.

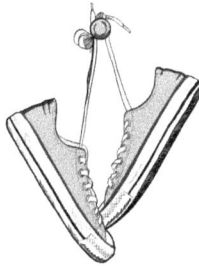

About the Author

MELISSA WOGAHN is a National Board Certified Health & Wellness Coach who loves working with people who hate to exercise. Melissa believes that everyone deserves to live their own active life so they can feel better, sleep better and live their best life.

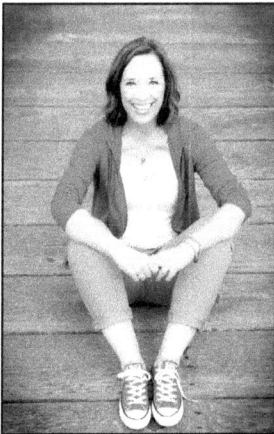

Melissa has developed health and fitness education programs for organizations including the *Los Angeles Times*, Good Samaritan Hospital and the American Heart Association. In addition, she provides fitness services for the County of San Diego. Melissa currently offers private and group health coaching programs. She enjoys speaking on all things related to living an active life.

In addition to being board certified, Melissa holds a master's degree in exercise physiology from the University of Southern California, is a Certified Strength and Conditioning Specialist and a credentialed provider for the American College of Sports Medicine's *Exercise is Medicine* initiative, a program aimed at connecting physicians with top health and fitness providers.

When not working, Melissa can be found walking her two cattle dogs, riding her vintage bicycle or dancing to her favorite R&B tunes.

Learn more at **JoyOfActiveLiving.com.**

Download additional, blank worksheets in PDF format at **JoyOfActiveLiving.com/couch.**

www.ingramcontent.com/pod-product-compliance
Lightning Source LLC
Chambersburg PA
CBHW071234020426
42333CB00015B/1472